FLU

101 FOR PREVENTING FLU

DR. J. SIMON

Contents

INTRODUCTION

Influenza, commonly known as the flu, is a contagious respiratory illness caused by influenza viruses. The flu can affect people of all ages and can lead to mild to severe symptoms. It is characterized by the sudden onset of symptoms and can result in seasonal outbreaks, often during the fall and winter months.

Key points about the flu include:

Viral Cause:

Influenza is caused by influenza viruses, specifically types A, B, and, less commonly, C. Influenza A and B viruses are responsible for seasonal flu outbreaks.

Transmission:

The flu is highly contagious and spreads through respiratory droplets when an infected person coughs, sneezes, or talks. It can also spread by touching a surface or object with the virus and then touching the face.

Symptoms:

Common symptoms of the flu include fever, chills, cough, sore throat, runny or stuffy nose, muscle or body aches, headaches, fatigue, and sometimes vomiting and diarrhea.

Seasonal Variability:

The flu is known for its seasonal variability, with peak activity typically occurring during the fall and winter months. Different strains of influenza viruses circulate each flu season.

Problems:

While most people recover from the flu without complications, it can lead to severe illness, particularly in high-risk groups such as young children, elderly individuals, pregnant women, and those with underlying health conditions.

Vaccination:

Annual flu vaccination is a key preventive measure. The flu vaccine is designed to protect against specific influenza strains expected to circulate during a given season.

Antiviral Medications:

Antiviral medications may be prescribed to treat the flu, especially in individuals at higher risk of complications or those with severe symptoms. These medications work best when started early in the course of the illness.

Preventive Measures:

Practicing good hygiene, including frequent handwashing, covering coughs and sneezes, and avoiding close contact with sick individuals, can help prevent the spread of the flu.

Stay Home When Sick:

Individuals with flu-like symptoms should stay home to avoid spreading the virus to others. It is advisable to seek medical attention if symptoms are severe or persistent.

Monitoring for Complications:

Individuals, especially those in high-risk groups, should monitor for signs of severe illness and seek prompt medical attention if complications are suspected.

The flu can have a significant impact on public health, leading to hospitalizations and, in some cases, fatalities. Vaccination, along with preventive measures and prompt medical attention when needed, plays a crucial role in reducing the impact of the flu on individuals and communities.

CHAPTER ONE

Defining Influenza

The flu, short for influenza, is a viral infection caused by influenza viruses. It primarily affects the respiratory system and is characterized by the sudden onset of symptoms. Here are key definitions related to the flu:

Influenza:

Influenza, commonly known as the flu, is an infectious respiratory illness caused by influenza viruses. It can lead to a range of symptoms, from mild to severe, and is associated with seasonal outbreaks.

Influenza Viruses:

Influenza viruses belong to the Orthomyxoviridae family and are classified into three types: A, B, and C. Influenza A and B viruses are responsible for seasonal flu outbreaks, while Influenza C viruses cause milder respiratory infections.

Seasonal Flu:

The seasonal flu refers to the annual occurrence of influenza outbreaks, typically during the fall and winter months. Different strains of influenza viruses circulate each flu season.

Symptoms of the Flu:

Common symptoms of the flu include fever, chills, cough, sore throat, runny or stuffy nose, muscle or body aches, headaches, fatigue, and sometimes vomiting and diarrhea.

Respiratory Droplets:

The flu is highly contagious and primarily spreads through respiratory droplets produced when an infected person coughs, sneezes, or talks. It can also spread by touching surfaces or objects with the virus and then touching the face.

Problems:

While most individuals recover from the flu without complications, it can lead to severe illness, especially in high-risk groups such as young children, elderly individuals, pregnant women, and those with underlying health conditions.

Flu Vaccine:

The flu vaccine is an annual preventive measure designed to protect against specific influenza strains expected to circulate during a given flu season. It is recommended for individuals aged six months and older.

Antiviral Medications:

Antiviral medications, such as oseltamivir (Tamiflu) and zanamivir (Relenza), may be prescribed to treat the flu, especially in individuals at higher risk of complications or those with severe symptoms.

Hygiene Practices:

Good hygiene practices, including frequent handwashing, covering coughs and sneezes, and avoiding close contact with sick individuals, help prevent the spread of the flu.

Flu-Like Illness:

Flu-like illness refers to a set of symptoms that resemble those of the flu but may be caused by other respiratory viruses. Influenza testing is often needed to confirm a diagnosis of the flu.

Understanding these definitions can contribute to better awareness, prevention, and management of the flu, a contagious respiratory infection that affects millions of individuals worldwide each year.

Influenza viruses are classified into three main types: A, B, and C. These types are further divided into different strains based on their surface proteins, hemagglutinin (H) and neuraminidase (N). The classification is based on the genetic makeup of the viruses and helps in monitoring and responding to flu outbreaks. Here are the main types and some notable strains of influenza:

Influenza Type A (H1N1 and H3N2):

Influenza A viruses are the most common and have the broadest host range, infecting humans, birds, and other animals. Notable strains include:

H1N1: Responsible for the 1918 Spanish flu pandemic and the 2009 H1N1 pandemic.

H3N2: Associated with seasonal flu outbreaks and can cause more severe illness, especially in older adults.

Influenza Type B:

Influenza B viruses primarily infect humans and cause seasonal flu. Unlike Type A, influenza B viruses are not classified into subtypes, but they are further divided into lineages and strains.

Influenza Type C:

Influenza C viruses cause mild respiratory infections and are less common than Types A and B. They do not cause seasonal flu outbreaks.

Influenza A Subtypes:

Influenza A viruses are further categorized based on their H and N proteins. For example, H5N1 and H7N9 are subtypes associated with avian influenza outbreaks. These subtypes may have the potential for causing severe human illness.

H1N1 Strains:

H1N1 strains have been responsible for various flu pandemics throughout history. The 2009 H1N1 pandemic, often referred to as "swine flu," was caused by a novel H1N1 strain that emerged in humans.

H3N2 Strains:

H3N2 strains are associated with seasonal flu and can lead to more severe illness, especially in older individuals. Different H3N2 strains circulate each flu season.

B/Victoria and B/Yamagata Lineages:

Influenza B viruses are divided into two lineages: B/Victoria and B/Yamagata. Both lineages can co-circulate during a flu season. The quadrivalent flu vaccine typically includes strains from both lineages.

Avian Influenza Strains:

Certain influenza A strains primarily infect birds but have the potential to infect humans. Notable examples include H5N1 (bird flu) and H7N9. These strains can cause severe illness and have been associated with outbreaks in poultry.

It's important to note that the flu viruses undergo regular genetic changes through antigenic drift, leading to the emergence of new strains. This variability requires ongoing surveillance and the development of updated flu vaccines each year to match the circulating strains and provide effective protection. The World Health Organization (WHO) monitors flu activity globally and recommends the composition of seasonal flu vaccines based on the predominant strains.

Signs and symptoms

The symptoms of the flu, or influenza, can vary in severity but generally manifest suddenly. Flu symptoms can affect the respiratory system and the entire body. Typical signs and symptoms include of:

Fever:

A sudden onset of high fever is a hallmark symptom of the flu. Fever is often one of the first signs of infection.

Chills:

Many individuals with the flu experience chills, which can accompany fever.

Cough:

A persistent and dry cough is a common flu symptom. It can be accompanied by chest discomfort.

Sore Throat:

A sore throat is often present and can contribute to discomfort, making swallowing painful.

Runny or Stuffy Nose:

Nasal congestion, runny nose, and sneezing are common flu symptoms, although they may be less prominent than with the common cold.

Muscle or Body Aches:

Severe muscle aches and body pains, often described as feeling like you've been hit by a truck, are common flu symptoms.

Headache:

Headaches are a frequent symptom of the flu and can range from mild to severe.

Fatigue:

Profound fatigue and weakness are common during the flu. Individuals may feel exhausted and lack energy.

Vomiting and Diarrhea (more common in children):

Some individuals, particularly children, may experience vomiting and diarrhea. These symptoms are less common in adults.

Difficulty Breathing or Shortness of Breath:

In severe cases, the flu can lead to respiratory symptoms such as difficulty breathing or shortness of breath. This may be more common in individuals with underlying respiratory conditions.

It's important to note that the symptoms of the flu can overlap with those of other respiratory infections, such as the common cold or respiratory syncytial virus (RSV). However, the sudden onset of severe symptoms, including high fever and body aches, is more characteristic of the flu.

Individuals experiencing flu-like symptoms, especially those at higher risk of complications, should seek medical attention promptly. Antiviral medications may be prescribed to reduce the severity and duration of symptoms, particularly if started early in the course of the illness. Additionally, staying hydrated, getting plenty of rest, and practicing good respiratory hygiene can help manage flu symptoms and support recovery.

The flu, or influenza, is highly contagious and primarily spreads through respiratory droplets produced when an infected person talks, coughs, or sneezes. The transmission of the flu involves several key factors:

Respiratory Droplets:

When an infected person talks, coughs, or sneezes, respiratory droplets containing the influenza virus are released into the air. These droplets can travel a short distance and land in the mouths or noses of people nearby.

Airborne Transmission:

In certain situations, particularly in enclosed spaces or crowded settings, respiratory droplets containing the flu virus can become aerosolized and remain in the air for a longer period. This can increase the risk of airborne transmission to individuals in the vicinity.

Contact with Contaminated Surfaces:

The flu virus can also spread by touching surfaces or objects contaminated with respiratory droplets and then touching the face, especially the mouth, nose, or eyes. This highlights the importance of practicing good hand hygiene to prevent transmission.

CHAPTER TWO

Direct Contact:

Direct contact with an infected person, such as hugging or shaking hands, can facilitate the transmission of the flu. Close contact with someone who has the flu increases the risk of exposure.

Asymptomatic Transmission:

Some individuals infected with the flu may not exhibit symptoms (asymptomatic carriers) but can still spread the virus to others. This makes it challenging to identify and isolate individuals who may be contagious.

Contagious Period:

People with the flu are typically most contagious in the first three to four days after the onset of symptoms. However, individuals can remain contagious for up to a week or longer, especially in children and individuals with weakened immune systems.

Pre-symptomatic Transmission:

Individuals infected with the flu can transmit the virus to others before they show symptoms (pre-symptomatic transmission). This adds complexity to efforts to prevent the spread of the virus.

Given the contagious nature of the flu, preventive measures are crucial to reducing transmission. These measures include:

Flu Vaccination:

Annual flu vaccination is a key preventive measure to protect against specific influenza strains and reduce the severity of illness.

Good Respiratory Hygiene:

Covering the mouth and nose when coughing or sneezing helps prevent the release of respiratory droplets. Using tissues or the elbow to cover the mouth is recommended.

Hand Hygiene:

Frequent handwashing with soap and water for at least 20 seconds, or using alcohol-based hand sanitizers, helps prevent the spread of the virus from contaminated surfaces to the face.

Avoiding Close Contact:

Avoid close contact with individuals who have the flu, especially during the contagious period.

Staying Home When Sick:

Individuals with flu-like symptoms should stay home to prevent the spread of the virus to others.

By implementing these preventive measures, individuals can contribute to reducing the transmission of the flu within communities and minimizing the impact of seasonal outbreaks.

Diagnosis and Testing

The diagnosis of influenza, or the flu, is typically based on clinical evaluation and may involve laboratory testing in certain cases. Key aspects of the diagnosis and testing process for the flu include:

Clinical Assessment:

Healthcare providers often begin the diagnostic process by conducting a thorough clinical evaluation. They inquire about the patient's symptoms, medical history, and recent exposure to individuals with flu-like symptoms.

Rapid Influenza Diagnostic Tests (RIDTs):

Rapid influenza diagnostic tests (RIDTs) are commonly used in healthcare settings to quickly detect the presence of influenza viruses. These tests can provide results within approximately 15-30 minutes.

Polymerase Chain Reaction (PCR) Testing:

Polymerase chain reaction (PCR) testing is a more sensitive and specific method for diagnosing the flu. It detects the genetic material of the influenza virus and can distinguish between different influenza types and subtypes.

Nucleic Acid Amplification Tests (NAATs):

NAATs, including PCR, are molecular diagnostic tests that amplify and detect the genetic material of the influenza virus. These tests are highly sensitive and can identify specific strains of the virus.

Viral Culture:

Viral culture involves growing influenza viruses from respiratory specimens collected from the patient. While less commonly used due to the time-consuming nature of the process, viral culture provides information about the infecting virus and its characteristics.

Serological Testing:

Serological testing involves measuring the levels of antibodies specific to influenza viruses in a patient's blood. While not commonly used for routine diagnosis, serological testing can be helpful for surveillance and research purposes.

Point-of-Care Testing:

In addition to RIDTs, some healthcare settings may use point-of-care testing methods that provide rapid results. These tests are designed to be performed at the point of care, such as in a doctor's office or clinic.

It's important to note that the accuracy of diagnostic tests may vary, and false-negative results can occur. Clinical judgment, based on symptoms and exposure history, plays a crucial role in the diagnosis of the flu.

During flu seasons or outbreaks, healthcare providers may rely on a combination of clinical assessment and testing to promptly diagnose and initiate appropriate management. Antiviral medications may be prescribed, especially if started early in the course of the illness.

For individuals with severe respiratory symptoms or those at higher risk of complications, healthcare providers may conduct diagnostic testing to guide treatment decisions and help prevent the spread of the virus.

<h2 style="text-align:center">Methods of Therapy</h2>

The treatment of influenza (flu) involves a combination of supportive care, antiviral medications, and preventive measures. The goals of treatment are to alleviate symptoms, reduce the severity and duration of illness, and prevent complications. Here are key approaches to treating the flu:

Antiviral Medications:

Antiviral medications are prescription drugs that can be effective in treating the flu, especially when initiated early in the course of the illness.

The two main classes of antiviral drugs used for influenza treatment are neuraminidase inhibitors:

- Oseltamivir (Tamiflu): Taken orally.
- Zanamivir (Relenza): Administered via inhalation.

Antiviral medications are most beneficial when started within 48 hours of the onset of symptoms. They can help reduce the severity and duration of illness, lessen the risk of complications, and shorten the duration of viral shedding.

Supportive Care:

Supportive care aims to alleviate symptoms and promote comfort during the recovery process. Key supportive measures include:

Rest: Get plenty of rest to allow the body to recover.

Hydration: Drink fluids such as water, herbal teas, and clear broths to stay hydrated.

Pain Relievers: Over-the-counter pain relievers, such as acetaminophen (Tylenol) or ibuprofen (Advil, Motrin), can help reduce fever, muscle aches, and headaches. Follow recommended dosages.

Fever Management:

Managing fever is an important aspect of flu treatment. Use appropriate fever-reducing medications and consider using cool compresses or taking a lukewarm bath.

Respiratory Support:

For individuals with respiratory symptoms, using a humidifier or taking steamy showers can help ease congestion and throat discomfort. Cough medications may be considered based on individual symptoms.

Isolation and Preventive Measures:

Individuals with the flu should isolate themselves to prevent the spread of the virus to others. Practice good respiratory hygiene, including covering the mouth and nose when coughing or sneezing, and frequently washing hands.

Follow Healthcare Provider Recommendations:

Follow the recommendations and prescribed treatments provided by healthcare providers. If antiviral medications are prescribed, complete the full course even if symptoms improve before finishing the medication.

It's important to note that antibiotics are not effective against viral infections like the flu. Antibiotics target bacterial infections, and the flu is caused by influenza viruses.

Individuals at higher risk of flu-related complications, such as young children, elderly individuals, pregnant women, and those with underlying health conditions, should seek medical attention promptly. Antiviral medications may be particularly beneficial for these individuals to reduce the risk of severe outcomes.

Preventive measures, including annual flu vaccination, play a key role in reducing the risk of influenza infection and minimizing the impact of seasonal outbreaks.

Preventive Strategies

Preventive strategies for influenza (flu) are crucial in reducing the risk of infection and minimizing the impact of seasonal outbreaks. Here are key preventive measures individuals can take to protect themselves and others from the flu:

Annual Flu Vaccination:

Receive the annual flu vaccine, which is designed to provide protection against specific influenza strains expected to circulate during the flu season. Vaccination is recommended for individuals aged six months and older.

Good Respiratory Hygiene:

Practice good respiratory hygiene to prevent the spread of respiratory droplets:

Cover the mouth and nose with a tissue or the elbow when coughing or sneezing.

Dispose of used tissues properly.

Frequent Handwashing:

Wash hands frequently with soap and water for at least 20 seconds, especially after coughing, sneezing, or being in public places. Use alcohol-based hand sanitizers if soap and water are not available.

Avoid Touching the Face:

Avoid touching the face, especially the mouth, nose, and eyes, to reduce the risk of introducing the virus into the body.

Avoiding Close Contact:

Minimize close contact with individuals who have flu-like symptoms, and practice physical distancing when possible.

CHAPTER THREE

Staying Home When Sick:

If you have flu-like symptoms, stay home to prevent the spread of the virus to others. This includes staying home from work, school, and social gatherings.

Environmental Hygiene:

Regularly clean and disinfect frequently-touched surfaces, such as doorknobs, light switches, and shared electronic devices, to reduce the risk of surface transmission.

Wearing Masks in Public:

In situations where flu activity is high or during outbreaks, wearing masks in public places may be recommended to reduce the transmission of respiratory droplets.

Promoting Vaccination in High-Risk Groups:

Encourage flu vaccination, especially among high-risk groups such as young children, elderly individuals, pregnant women, and those with underlying health conditions.

Educating and Raising Awareness:

Educate individuals and communities about the importance of flu prevention, vaccination, and recognizing flu symptoms. Promote awareness through public health campaigns.

Maintaining a Healthy Lifestyle:

Adopting a healthy lifestyle, including regular exercise, a balanced diet, adequate sleep, and stress management, can support overall immune system function.

It's important to note that these preventive strategies are most effective when implemented collectively at the community level. Public health initiatives, such as vaccination campaigns and awareness programs, play a crucial role in reducing the overall impact of influenza on public health. Individuals should consult with healthcare providers for personalized guidance on flu prevention, especially if they belong to high-risk groups.

High-Risk Groups and Complications

Certain individuals are considered high-risk for complications associated with influenza (flu). High-risk groups are more susceptible to severe illness and complications if they contract the flu. Common high-risk groups include:

Young Children:

Children, especially those under the age of 5, are at an increased risk of flu-related complications. This includes infants and toddlers.

Elderly Individuals:

Adults aged 65 and older are more vulnerable to severe outcomes and complications from the flu. The immune response may weaken with age.

Pregnant Women:

Pregnant women are at an increased risk of complications due to changes in the immune and respiratory systems. Flu infection during pregnancy can also impact the health of the unborn child.

Individuals with Chronic Health Conditions:

People with underlying health conditions, such as:

- Chronic lung diseases (e.g., asthma, chronic obstructive pulmonary disease - COPD).
- Heart disease.
- Diabetes.
- Kidney disorders.
- Liver disorders.

- Neurological conditions.

- Weakened immune systems (e.g., due to medications or diseases like HIV/AIDS).

Residents of Long-Term Care Facilities:

Individuals residing in long-term care facilities, such as nursing homes and assisted living facilities, are at an increased risk of flu-related complications due to close living quarters and shared spaces.

American Indian and Alaska Native Populations:

Certain racial and ethnic groups, including American Indian and Alaska Native populations, may have an elevated risk of flu-related complications.

Complications of the flu can include:

Pneumonia:

Influenza can lead to viral or bacterial pneumonia, which is a serious respiratory infection affecting the lungs.

Bronchitis and Sinus Infections:

Flu can contribute to the development of bronchitis and sinus infections, particularly in individuals with pre-existing respiratory conditions.

Exacerbation of Chronic Health Conditions:

The flu can worsen existing chronic health conditions, such as heart disease, diabetes, and asthma.

Ear Infections:

In children, the flu may lead to ear infections, which can be painful and may require medical attention.

Dehydration:

Fever, vomiting, and diarrhea associated with the flu can lead to dehydration, especially in young children and older adults.

Neurological Complications:

In rare cases, influenza can lead to neurological complications, such as encephalitis (inflammation of the brain) or seizures.

Given the increased risk of complications, individuals in high-risk groups are strongly encouraged to receive the annual flu vaccine and seek prompt medical attention if flu-like symptoms develop. Healthcare providers may consider antiviral medications to reduce the severity and duration of symptoms, especially when initiated early in the course of the illness. Preventive measures, such as good respiratory hygiene and staying home when sick, are crucial for protecting high-risk individuals from flu exposure.

CONCLUSION

In conclusion, influenza, or the flu, is a contagious respiratory illness caused by influenza viruses. It poses a significant public health concern, leading to seasonal outbreaks and occasional pandemics. Understanding the symptoms, transmission, and preventive strategies is crucial for individuals and communities.

Key points about the flu include:

Symptoms: The flu is characterized by symptoms such as fever, cough, sore throat, body aches, fatigue, and respiratory symptoms. It can range from mild to severe, and certain individuals are at a higher risk of complications.

Transmission: The flu primarily spreads through respiratory droplets produced when an infected person talks, coughs, or sneezes. It can also spread by touching contaminated surfaces and then touching the face.

Prevention: Annual flu vaccination is a highly effective preventive measure. Good respiratory hygiene, frequent handwashing, avoiding close contact with sick individuals, and staying home when sick are essential preventive strategies.

High-Risk Groups: Certain individuals, including young children, elderly individuals, pregnant women, and those with chronic health conditions, are considered high-risk for flu-related complications. Vaccination is particularly important for these groups.

Complications: Complications of the flu can include pneumonia, bronchitis, exacerbation of chronic health conditions, and neurological complications. High-risk individuals are more susceptible to severe outcomes.

Treatment: Antiviral medications can be prescribed to reduce the severity and duration of flu symptoms, especially when initiated early. Supportive care, including rest, hydration, and fever management, is also important.

Preventive Strategies: In addition to vaccination, preventive strategies include practicing good respiratory and hand hygiene, avoiding close contact with sick individuals, and promoting awareness in communities.

Flu prevention is a collective effort that involves individuals, healthcare providers, and public health initiatives. By staying informed, getting vaccinated, and adopting preventive measures, individuals can contribute to reducing the impact of the flu on public health. Seeking prompt medical attention and following healthcare provider recommendations are crucial, especially for high-risk individuals.

THE END